Why do so many people struggle with weight in our society when the vast majority in other cultures never seem to grow fat? What causes the distortions to our bodies, not only in body size and fat deposits, but also in our biochemistry? Is it really weakness of character or lack of willpower that makes us eat too much and gain weight? And—most important of all—is there a way of eating and living so that whatever distortions have already appeared will disappear quite naturally as part of the process of regenerating the body through food and exercise? The answer is "Yes!" You can lose fat—but only if you understand why most diets don't work.

By Leslie Kenton
Published by Ivy Books:

BEAT STRESS
BOOST ENERGY
GET FIT
LOOK GREAT
LOSE FAT
SLEEP DEEP

LOSE FAT

Leslie Kenton

IVY BOOKS • NEW YORK

Ivy Books
Published by Ballantine Books
Copyright © 1996 by Leslie Kenton

http://www.randomhouse.com

Library of Congress Catalog Card Number: 96-94971

ISBN 0-8041-1624-5

Manufactured in the United States of America

First American Edition: March 1997

10   9   8   7   6   5   4   3   2   1

Contents

Author's Note

The material in this book is intended for information purposes only. None of the suggestions or information is meant to be prescriptive. Any attempt to treat a medical condition should always come under the directions of a competent physician. Readers should always consult with a health care professional before starting a new diet or exercise program. Neither the publisher nor I can accept responsibility for injuries or illness arising out of a failure by a reader to take medical advice. I am only a reporter. I also have a profound interest in helping myself and others maximize our potential for positive health.

LOSE FAT

CHAPTER 1

Let Diets Die

Why Diets Don't Work

Why do so many people struggle with weight in our society when the vast majority in other cultures never seem to grow fat? What causes the distortions to our bodies, not only in body size and fat deposits, but also in our biochemistry? Is it really weakness of character or lack of willpower that makes us eat too much and gain weight? And—most important of all—is there a way of eating and living so that whatever distortions have already appeared will disappear quite naturally as part of the process of regenerating the body through food and exercise? The answer is "Yes!" You can lose fat—but only if you understand why most diets don't work.

What it means to be lean

To be lean means to have a low percentage of *body fat*. A lean body is always smaller in size than a thin body of the same weight since muscle tissue is much denser than fat tissue. Get lean and you gain enormously in energy, stamina, and general health. You can also end up looking years younger. And where you once had to watch every calorie you consumed in order not to gain weight, you will be able to eat without worrying about calories. The sad truth is that slicing calories off your daily menus does not necessarily shave padding from your hips. The human body has far too complex a system of defenses designed to protect its fat stores.

Why do we often feel only half alive? The key to vitality is found in the body itself. It lies in the same place as the key to burning excess fat—in muscle. Your muscle is the engine that turns food calories into energy, burns fat, and creates an experience of ongoing simple joy. Muscle creates the life-energy for you to think, to move, and to feel.

Animal bodies, like ours, are made up of two basic components: *lean body mass* (LBM), which encompasses our muscle tissue, and *fat*. Lean body mass—the part that is not fat—is the part of you that is most alive. It consists of your organs such as the heart, the liver, the pancreas; your bones and skin; and your muscle tissue. The hardest thing for most of us who have been brainwashed by low-calorie dieting nonsense to understand is that it is your body's *fat* stores that are the enemy, not your weight as measured by the scales.

Fat tissue is very different from your muscle. It does not need oxygen, does not create movement or activity, and cannot repair itself.

The yo–yo effect

Stick to a calorie-restricted diet for a few weeks and you get thinner. But when you resume your old eating habits, the weight you lost begins to creep back on. Sooner or later this regain leads you to try dieting again and what is known as the *yo-yo effect* comes about. But each time you shed pounds, they are drawn from both your body's fat stores *and* its muscle stores. However, each time you regain it, it comes back as *fat*.

Every dieting regime that reduces the body's

muscle stock is doomed to failure. For it is only in muscle cells that fat is burned.

Let diets die

Some popular diets are nutritionally inadequate to a degree that in the long run they not only contribute to weight *gain* instead of permanent fat loss but can also do serious damage to your body and to your looks.

The Lose Fat scheme has two elements—nutrition and exercise—and is designed to help you to live longer and better while your body slowly and inexorably transforms its shape.

"Go Primitive" nutrition

The Go Primitive diet is the nutritional side of the Lose Fat scheme. It is based on what I call *real foods*—beans, fruits, vegetables, whole grains such as brown rice, wheat, rye, barley, millet, quinoa, and leafy and root vegetables. A way of eating that is low in fats, refined starches, and sugars, moderate in protein and rich in fiber, and high in complex carbohydrates from natural foods, it asks that, as much as you can, you choose foods grown on healthy soils and eat them in a form as close as possible to their natural state, either cooked or raw.

Exercise and grow lean

The second element of the Lose Fat scheme is exercise. Body fat is only burned within a crucible of muscle, in the presence of both carbohydrate and oxygen. The right kind of exercise for fat loss and permanent weight control both increases lean body mass by building and enhancing metabolism and brings oxygen in good supply to the muscle cells where fat is burned.

Losing fat this way is a slow and completely transformative process—slow because it is organic, that is, regulated from within by your own individual metabolism. This makes shedding excess weight safe, effective, and lasting. It is designed to dispose only of excess body fat while protecting your muscles and your body water. Such a process has to be slow so that your body is protected from cannibalizing its own muscle tissue and so that fat retention survival mechanisms are not triggered to defeat you in the accomplishment of your goal.

DO IT NOW

- Decide now to *let diets die* forever.

- Forget about every diet food and appetite suppressant you ever heard of.

- Stop counting calories.

- Decide that *you* matter. Commit yourself to doing whatever is in your power week by week to enhance your health and energy while you grow lean.

CHAPTER 2

Go Primitive

Unnatural Food

A lot has happened to our foods in the last century. First, they are *grown* differently from the way our ancestors grew theirs for thousands of years. We grow food on chemically fertilized soils in which the organic matter has been degraded or destroyed. Eating foods grown in this way leads to depletion and imbalance in minerals and trace elements—both of which we need in good quantities to support complex metabolic processes on which health and leanness depend. Secondly, our foods are now highly *processed*. Raw foodstuffs, instead of being

made into meals in home kitchens as they
were earlier this century, are sent to food
manufacturers where they are fragmented—
literally broken apart physically and chemically—then put through complex processes to
alter them out of all recognition. Thirdly, our
foods are shipped over long distances and
stored for long periods of time, which lowers
their nutritional value.

Back to nature

Our forebears ate foods that were little processed: these foods were *eaten whole, as close
as possible to their natural state*. Also, they ate
meat rarely, and usually only sparingly.

Returning to what I call a Go Primitive way
of eating can help you lose fat and restore
normal weight even to people who are very
overweight. It can also free you from much suf-
fering caused by degenerative conditions such
as high blood pressure, arteriosclerosis, diabetes, and other Western diseases.

Go Primitive is primarily *vegan*—a vegetarian way of eating that excludes dairy
products such as milk, cheese, yogurt, and
eggs. This is because, like meat, all of these
foods tend to be high in fat and fat is the one
kind of food that you need very little of while

getting rid of your own fat deposits. But Go Primitive does not *have* to be vegetarian. If you feel you *must* eat meat or fish by all means have them—but *occasionally*, or in small quantities, instead of as big main courses. And choose meats and fish wisely from ultra-lean, clean sources. Eat venison, for instance, or free-range boar, wild cod, and wild pollack instead of beef, lamb, farmed salmon, and ordinary pork.

DO IT NOW

- Right now forgive yourself for any past "failures" in weight control. They are *not* your fault.

   You are not weak-willed or hopeless. You have only been caught in a lose-lose scenario.

- Decide to explore the Go Primitive raw materials and begin to experiment with them. It is a whole new world.

- Go organic wherever possible when buying grains and legumes, vegetables and fruits.

- Find out more about pesticide control in

> your area and put pressure on the gov-
> ernment to improve things.
>
> · Stop buying highly processed foods.

Quickstart

Go Primitive has two phases. The first phase, Quickstart, is *ultra-low in fat.* It is designed specifically to be used during the period in which your body's excess fat deposits are being shed. During this phase only 10–15 percent of your calories are taken in as fat. Quickstart has no cholesterol (unless you choose to eat small quantities of milk, eggs, and meat products), is high in fiber, and excludes nuts, olives, avocados, and all but the smallest quantities of high-fat seeds.

Every gram of fat you eat has more than twice the calories of a gram of carbohydrate, and each fat calorie is harder to burn and easier to turn into body fat. High-fat foods also raise the level of cholesterol and uric acid in your tissues, paving the way for arteriosclerosis and gout. They also interfere with efficient carbohydrate metabolism and encourage blood-sugar disturbances that can lead to diabetes or a prediabetic state. Finally, fats in meat, fish, dairy products, oils, margarines, and butter are the foods that carry the highest concentrations of pollutants from pesticides and other chemicals.

Stop counting calories

Go Primitive does not restrict your calories, but most people using Quickstart, although they may eat twice the amount of food they have been used to, will actually consume far fewer calories than the average person on a typical Western diet. On a Go Primitive diet of natural foods high in complex carbohydrates you will lose weight without calorie counting until you reach your ideal weight.

It is essential that your body be supplied with quantities of complex carbohydrates and that you don't go hungry. Complex carbohydrates are the energy foods that sustain you throughout the day and protect you from the hunger that defeats dieters on calorie-restricted diets. But unless you get enough complex carbohydrates your body cannot burn fat properly.

COMPLEX CARBOHYDRATES

Here are the most important things to remember about complex carbohydrates.

- They are your main source of energy.

- Eating a diet high in complex carbohydrates protects your body's muscle stores and lets your body use its fat as energy.

- 60–75 percent of the calories you consume need to come from complex carbohydrates.

- The digestion of carbohydrates starts when food enters your mouth. If you don't chew well you don't digest carbohydrates properly and this can impede fat burning.

- When you eat a diet high in complex carbohydrates and low in fat (15–20 percent fat) your blood sugar remains stable. You gain natural appetite control and emotional stability.

Western Diet	Quickstart	Living Lean
25–50% carbohydrate (simple)	70–75% carbohydrate (complex)	50–75% carbohydrate (complex)
25% protein	15–20% protein	10–20% protein
40–50% fat	10–15% fat	20–25% fat

Proteins

Proteins both from foods and in your body are made up of building blocks called amino acids of which there are 22 different kinds. When you eat foods containing proteins your body breaks these proteins down into their constituent amino acids and with them reconstructs whatever new protein it needs. Whether you get your proteins from animal foods or vegetable foods makes not one bit of difference. One hundred years ago in the West two-thirds of our proteins came from plant foods, whereas now two-thirds come from animal foods. Although no single plant source apart from soy beans contains all the essential amino acids, a variety of plant foods will supply them all. There are a thousand ways of doing this (see the recipe section for some ideas to start you off).

On Go Primitive, making sure you get enough protein is something you do not have to think about at all as long as you eat some grains and some legumes during the day—ideally, approximately one-third legumes to two-thirds grains.

Living Lean

Living Lean is the second phase of Go Primitive. It differs from Quickstart only in that it is more liberal in the use of natural high-fat foods such as avocados, olives, nuts, and seeds. It aims for no more than 25 percent of your calories to be taken in fat.

Both Quickstart and Living Lean have many things in common. They

- do not restrict calories.

- are low in fat and have virtually no cholesterol.

- exclude most free fats (except a little olive oil or soy oil).

- are high in fiber.

- exclude caffeine and other stimulants.

- are based on real foods including whole fruits, vegetables, whole grains, and beans.

- exclude meat, fish, poultry, and milk products, except occasionally or as condiments.

- exclude all refined and processed oils and fat.

- exclude refined sugars and simple carbohydrates such as white bread and most packaged cereals.

- discourage the use of alcohol except occasionally, at a level of less than 60 ml (2 fl oz) of alcohol a day.

Fat Facts

Fats can be roughly divided into two groups—saturated and unsaturated. Saturated fats (found in meat, dairy products such as cheese,

ice cream, and milk, and tropical oils such as
palm kernel and coconut) are stable, inactive,
and virtually inert in your body. Their only
raison d'etre is to provide calories in a concentrated form that can later be burned as energy.
Unsaturated fats come in two forms: *mono-*
unsaturates such as olive oil, and *poly-*
unsaturates, found in corn, sunflower seeds,
peanuts, and many other foods from which
they are extracted. Monounsaturates and polyunsaturates are much more biologically active
—more able to easily take part in important
biochemical changes in your body that produce
energy, create hormones, and help burn stored
body fats.

Essential fatty acids

Your body can make all the fat it needs for
daily metabolic processes except for two essential fatty acids, *linoleic* and *linolenic*. They are
found naturally in fresh foods—in seeds and
nuts, in vegetables and fish—even in wild
meat such as game. For optimum health you
need no more than 2–4 tablespoons of these
essential fatty acids a day, yet, despite our
high fat intake in the West, they are hard to
find in modern convenience foods.

These two unsaturates play a vital role.

They help you burn body fat and build energy. Linoleic and linolenic are called essential fatty acids because that is exactly what they are—essential to human life and health. Important for your brain and nerve cells, your skin and hair, they also form the building blocks for cell membranes all over your body.

Free fats

The moment you remove an unsaturated fat from the food in which it comes you produce what is known as a *free fat*. A free fat is any fat that has been separated out from the food in which it occurs in nature—corn oil for instance, peanut or ground-nut oil, sunflower oil, safflower oil, and all the rest, as well as any margarines or biscuits or other foods containing them. Free fats are something to avoid like the plague, for through complex operations involving the use of heat and chemical solvents, food manufacturers turn our natural fatty acids into highly artificial fat products that can damage our health and impede weight loss.

As far as the golden vegetable oils that you find on supermarket shelves are concerned, don't use them. On your salads, instead of using salad oils, explore some of the recipes for

low-fat dressings or use a teaspoon or so of
cold-pressed extra virgin olive oil.

FAT CONTENT OF VARIOUS TYPES OF FOOD

Food group	Fat content
Grains, beans, fruits, and vegetables	0–15%
Low-fat fish	0–30%
Fatty fish (e.g., trout, mackerel, salmon)	50–60%
Milk	50%
Eggs and cheese	60–80%
Meat	60–85%

Polyunsaturates and hydrogenated oil

Not one mass-produced margarine on the
market is genuinely health-promoting despite
all the advertising to the contrary. Nor are all
those golden oils, salad dressings and biscuits,
breads or ready-made meals that contain
them. So don't be misled by the words *contains
polyunsaturates*. Margarines and cooking oils
are junk fats. Your body cannot use them

for health and their presence actually blocks the uptake of fatty acids in your diet. Even the ordinary saturated fat that you find in steak or chicken is healthier than such artificially produced, hydrogenated, unnatural fatty acids. It is important when shopping that you read every label: Leave on the shelf anything that says it contains hydrogenated vegetable oil.

DO IT NOW

- Go low fat.

- Use cold-pressed extra virgin olive oil and freshly ground flax seeds as your source of extra fatty acids.

- If you are not vegetarian, eat cold-water fish such as wild trout, wild salmon, mackerel, or sardines a couple of times a week.

- If you are vegetarian, sprinkle a tablespoon of freshly ground vacuum-packed linseeds or flax seeds each day on your cereals or salads or cooked dishes.

- Avoid *all* saturated fats.

- Avoid highly processed foods.

Vegetable fats v. animal fats

Essential fatty acids are found in abundance in
nuts, beans, grains, and seeds, as well as in
olives and other plant foods. With the excep-
tion of avocados, nuts, and olives, most of these
whole plant foods have a low fat content.
Animal foods, however, have a much higher
fat content, none of which you need for health
and all of which work against your developing
a lean body.

Liberate Your Energy

The key to shedding excess fat is *energy*: You
need to turn calories from your foods and
your fat stores into energy, while retaining
your muscle tissue and body water. Calorie-
restricted weight-loss diets don't do it. You
need to be sure about which kinds of foods to
eat and which to avoid. Finally, you need to
know how to protect yourself against blood-
sugar problems and insulin resistance (more
about this in a moment), both of which upset
appetite-control mechanisms and prevent your
fat stores from being burned.

Banish sugar bondage

The kind of food you eat matters, too. Carbohydrates are your body's main source of energy for all its functions, including fat burning. Getting enough complex carbohydrates prevents your body from using muscle as a source of energy and lets it use stored body fat instead. However, just any old carbohydrate won't do, only *complex* carbohydrates will—lots of unrefined grains. Complex carbohydrates both *spare muscle tissue* and *bring natural appetite control.*

One of the major weight-control problems caused by eating processed foods full of *simple* carbohydrates such as white flour and sugar is that it brings about a progressive decline in your body's ability to metabolize sugar. Unlike real foods full of protective fiber, refined and processed foods are highly concentrated foods. Fiber is no longer present to dilute their concentration and to slow down the rate at which the simple starches and sugars they contain are absorbed into your bloodstream. Continue to eat concentrated processed foods year after year and your blood-glucose levels will tend to get higher and higher as the pancreas is continually forced to release more and more insulin in an attempt to control it all.

Even though insulin is still being produced in high concentrations your body may become insulin resistant so that your cells no longer respond and the ability to control blood sugar is lost. When this happens, the calories from your foods are more and more easily converted into fats, which are then laid down as fat stores on your belly, hips, thighs, and bottom. You have also increased the likelihood of getting heart disease or other degenerative conditions, for insulin resistance is a phenomenon linked to arteriosclerosis as well as adult-onset diabetes.

The beans and lentils, grains, vegetables, and fruits of Go Primitive can save the day. Eating them helps stabilize blood sugar. Because these foods are high in fiber, real foods provide you with a steady stream of energy over many hours and prevent insulin resistance. The fiber they contain plays several other important roles in weight loss, too.

More than bran

Dietary fiber is an integral part of every vegetable food as it appears in nature. Fiber plays a central role both in weight loss and in the successful maintenance of normal weight. The naturally high-fiber Go Primitive diet of our ancestors had a low calorie density. People eating this way reach satiety far quicker than those munching away on the products of the Western food industry with their very *high* caloric density, devoid as they are of fiber and stuffed with junk fats and hidden sugars.

Deep cleansing

Fiber also helps keep your body clean. When wastes are allowed to build up in your system they can interfere with fat-burning energy production and also help to create false appetite. Natural high-fiber foods continually detoxify your body.

DO IT NOW

- Steer clear of *simple* carbohydrates—white flour and sugar.

- Eat plenty of *complex* carbohydrates—grains, beans, lentils, fruits, and vegetables.

- Throw out all those "fiber-enriched" breakfast cereals.

- Try to take in 40 grams of fiber a day from real foods.

GOOD SOURCES OF FIBER

You will find 10 grams of fiber in the following:

Fruits	**Weight**
Dried apricots	40g
Figs	50g
Dried prunes	60g
Nectarines	100g
Dates	114g
Black currants	115g
Raspberries	135g
Raisins	150g
Bananas	300g
Apples	400g
Pears	400g
Oranges	500g

Uncooked Grains	
Buckwheat	100g
Popcorn	100g
Oats	100g
Brown rice	230g
Barley	250g
Millet	300g
Wheat	400g

Beans, Peas, Lentils	Weight
Butter beans	36g
Green beans	40g
Kidney beans	40g
Mung beans	45g
Chickpeas	55g
Lentils	85g
Split peas	85g
Broad beans	160g
Adzuki beans	200g

Eat Early, Eat Slowly

There are two more unique features to the Lose Fat scheme. First is the way your meals are distributed, for it reverses the time when the major bulk of your foods are eaten. You are asked to eat breakfast like a king, lunch like a prince, and supper like a pauper. Second is the way the scheme asks for periods of rest *between* meals. Clinical experience shows that not snacking or drinking anything except water between meals can improve digestion, help regulate blood sugar, and relieve the chronic hunger that so many dieters wrestle with.

Easy appetite control

One interesting fact about the appetite center
in the brain is that it takes twenty minutes
after you begin eating before this appetite
regulator can signal the stomach to turn off
your sense of appetite. Eat too fast and you
can easily swallow a lot more food than your
body really wants. It is important to eat slowly
and chew thoroughly. The flavor of foods comes
to you through chewing. Chewing plays a very
important part in satisfaction as well as in
digestion.

Digestive rhythms

Chewing is particularly important when it
comes to grains and cereals, beans and
legumes. The digestion of these complex carbohydrates begins in the mouth. If they are not
chewed thoroughly they will not be digested
properly and you can end up with indigestion
or flatulence.

The body does not digest foods effectively
and freely if you eat or drink anything but
water in between meals. Even nibbling a
handful of peanuts can delay digestion so
much so that 11 hours after breakfast there is

still a large residue of your meal sitting in your stomach.

DO IT NOW

- Always eat a good hearty breakfast.

- Decide to drink water between meals—lots of it.

- Explore the taste and textures of low-fat real foods by eating your fill of them without worrying about weight.

- Experiment with decreasing the size of your evening meal and see how it makes you feel.

- Read food labels carefully before you decide what to buy.

Every time we take new food into our mouth we stimulate our digestive juices. If we do this only a few hours after eating while our stomach is still engaged in the digestion of that meal, it is forced to turn its attention to the new food and begin the process all over again. It never gets a rest. Your stomach needs regular periods of rest, for digestion is highly demanding work.

The Lean Manifesto

If a Go Primitive way of eating is brand new to you, the best way to get into it is through small progressive changes, day by day and week by week. If you are a big meat eater begin by reducing the amount of meat you eat and choose only the leanest types to have twice a week, then cut down to perhaps once a week or once every two weeks until you let it dwindle to practically nothing. You can do the same with fish and milk products.

Be creative

The vegetables, dried beans, and grains that are the backbone of this kind of eating have superb colors and textures. Experiment with them but remember to introduce them slowly into whatever diet you have been used to. This is for two reasons. First, changing your diet dramatically in any direction can cause digestive upset because the human body tends to rebel against whatever it is not accustomed to. This is particularly important when introducing beans, peas, and lentils into your life. The balance of intestinal flora varies tremendously with the kind of foods you are used to.

Let them rebalance a bit before bombarding yourself with piles of beans. The second and more important reason to ease into Go Primitive is that the changes that are made slowly are the changes that *last*. Begin by making one meal a day on Go Primitive principles and notice how much better you feel in a week or two.

A note on alcohol

Concentrated and quickly absorbed, alcohol is not only easily transformed into fat within your body, it also tends to disturb the blood-sugar curve and unsettle the appetite. Have a drink and false appetite often appears within minutes, urging you to eat more than your body really wants. Also, alcohol is toxic to a number of the organs in the body.

Keep a checklist

Although you never need to count calories on Go Primitive, you will want to read labels carefully on any commercially prepared products to make sure that they fall well within the fat range of 10–15 percent during the Quickstart phase and 20–25 percent during Living Lean.

It is also a very good idea to keep a checklist day by day.

For recipes and helpers for the Go Primitive way of eating, go to the last chapter.

CHAPTER 3

Drink Yourself Lean

Only Water Works

Water is the most important nutrient of all. It is the stuff from which your blood, your cells, your muscles—even your bones—are mostly made. A healthy person who weighs 143 pounds carries about 42 quarts of water around—26 quarts inside the cells, almost 16 quarts outside, including 5 quarts in the blood. Let yourself become dehydrated and the chemical reactions in the cells involved in fat burning become sluggish. Your cells cannot build new tissue efficiently, toxic products

31

build up in your bloodstream, your blood
volume decreases so that you have less oxygen
and nutrients transported to your cells—all of
which are essential to fat burning. Dehydra-
tion also results in your feeling weak and tired
and can lead to overeating, as it disturbs
appetite mechanisms so you think you are
hungry even when you are not.

Water plays a major part in digesting your
food and absorbing nutrients, thanks to enzymes that are themselves mostly water. If you
fail to drink enough water between meals your
mouth becomes low in saliva and digestion suf-
fers. Water is also the medium through which
wastes are eliminated from your body. Each
time you exhale, you release highly humidified
air—about 2 big glasses' worth a day. Your kidneys and intestines eliminate another 6 or so
glasses every 24 hours, while another 2
glasses' worth are released through the pores
of your skin. That makes 10 glasses a day—
and this is on a *cool* day. When it gets hot,
when you are exercising, or when you are
working hard, the usual 10 glasses lost in this
way can triple.

Provided you do not suffer from a kidney or
liver disease, drinking 8 big glasses or more of
water a day not only helps you lose weight and

keep it off permanently, it improves the functioning of your whole body.

Hunger can be thirst

The control center for both thirst and hunger is in the same place in your body: the hypothalamus. Often when you think you are hungry what your body is trying to tell you is that you need to take in more water. Perhaps the best-kept secret in the world about weight control is this: Reach for a glass of water every time you feel hungry between meals and you will find your hunger diminishing within a few minutes. Try it and see.

There is another way in which drinking optimal quantities of water plays a central role in fat loss and weight control. It has to do with your kidneys. When some part of you needs more water, your kidneys make sure it arrives. Drinking lots of water—far more than you think you need—helps your kidneys to help your liver to help you lose weight.

Water is also the world's best natural diuretic. If your body tends to retain water this is often because you don't drink *enough* so it tries its best to hold on to the water there is. You need to cut out tea and coffee and drink much more water. Even if you have always been a committed 6 to 8 cups a day tea- or coffee-drinker, after a couple of weeks on good water you will find you don't miss it.

Many colas, sodas, and soft drinks contain caffeine and they are also far too high in sugar. They bring nutritionally empty calories into your body that you can ill afford, so cut them out.

DO IT NOW

- Cut down on and try to cut out coffee, tea, and all soft drinks.

- Divide your weight in pounds by 16, then round off the figure to discover how many 225 ml/8 oz glasses of water to drink each day.

- Drink two glasses of clean water on rising and then get your daily quota by drinking more between meals.

- When you are tempted to snack, reach for the water.

- Sit back and watch your energy increase.

Is pure water an illusion?

The quality of water you drink affects every biochemical reaction on which leanness depends. Take a good look at what inexpensive jug filters are available and start using one—for cooking, too. Be sure to change the filter it contains often and regularly. If you can afford it, use the best bottled water for drinking.

CHAPTER 4
===

Work Yourself Lean

Muscle Magic

What kind of exercise do you need for permanent weight control? Not the kind that goes all out to burn as many calories as possible. Far from it. That only *depletes* your energy, *slows* fat burning, and leaves you feeling exhausted and looking haggard. Exercise for fat loss needs to be slow, sustained, and regular, and it needs to do three things: enhance your metabolism, increase your supply of oxygen to the muscle cells for fat burning, and make the ratio of your lean body mass (LBM) to fat shift in favor of muscle. For this you need two kinds of exercise—*aerobic*, such as brisk walking, to stimulate oxygen supply, and *muscle-enhancing*, such as weight training.

Fat is dead

Because your body's fat tissues have a very low metabolic activity, they don't burn calories. Only your muscle cells do this. The more muscle tissue you have the better your body burns calories, sheds fat, and keeps it off. Also the more muscle you have the more you are able to eat without gaining weight. But you need a lot of oxygen to do this. Aerobic exercise enhances your body's oxygen transport and use. It could be running, walking, swimming, cycling, or any other activity that uses the large muscle groups and in which your heart beats steadily and you breathe deeply for a period of 20–45 minutes at least three, preferably four, times a week.

Body sculpture

To create for yourself a minimum exercise program, choose one of the following:

- walking 30–45 minutes 3 times a week (best of all for most people).

- cycling 40–45 minutes 3–5 times a week.

- jogging 30–45 minutes 3–5 times a week.

- rowing 30–45 minutes 3–5 times a week.

- swimming 30–45 minutes 3–5 times a week.

Exercise to build muscle, such as weight training using very light weights but many repetitions, is the most effective way of building LBM and uncovering your true body form. It chisels and defines arms, legs, torso, hips, and bottom, even if they have been neglected for many years and have lost their natural tone and shape.

Forget age

There is a widespread belief that as you get older your body metabolism naturally slows down and therefore you are less and less able to prevent yourself from becoming fat. Actually, age has absolutely nothing to do with it. It doesn't matter how old you are or how much you weigh now. What limits your ability to burn fat and stay lean is how long you have been inactive. It is long-term inactivity that wastes LBM and results in the muscle cells being unable to burn the calories.

Even if you have never tried any form of weight training before, you might enroll at a fitness center and give it a try.

DO IT NOW

- Start today to exercise.

- Find a friend and make a pact to exercise together 4 or 5 times a week.

- Experiment with different kinds of exercise to find out which you enjoy most. Enjoyment is an important factor in making exercise work for you.

- Make a note of how you feel on the days you do and don't exercise.

- Let yourself daydream about how your body will change in the next few months.

CHAPTER 5

Go for It—Go Primitive

Eat Your Fill

Go Primitive is based around two large meals a day—breakfast, which should supply between a third and a half of all the calories for the day, and a main meal, best eaten at lunchtime or at least before 4 o'clock in the afternoon if you can possibly manage it—with a very light meal in the evening. In between meals it is important to drink your quota of water. Begin with two

large glasses in the morning just as soon as
you get up, and then again throughout the
morning, afternoon, and evening until all you
intended to drink is finished. Always drink *between* meals since water can dilute substances
in the digestive system and interfere with the
efficiency of digestion and absorption. It is
important to reach for a glass or even two of
water whenever you happen to feel hungry
between meals. It is absolutely the best
appetite suppressant in the world.

Guidelines for Go Primitive

• Eat a big breakfast, a good main meal in the
  middle of the day, and the lightest of sup-
  pers, or no supper at all, preferably at least
  2 to 3 hours before going to bed.

• Avoid eating between meals since this slows
  the stomach from emptying, encourages food
  still in the stomach to ferment, and creates
  false appetite.

• Leave 5 hours between meals—to efficiently
  and completely digest the previous meal.

• Make mealtimes a pleasure. Eat slowly and
  chew your foods thoroughly so that you
  digest your foods properly, you don't end

up with digestive disturbances including intestinal gas, and you don't overeat.

- Drink lots of water—enough to make your urine quite pale—but always *between* meals. Give yourself 20 minutes water-free before a meal and half an hour afterward.

- Vary your foods from meal to meal, but don't eat too many different foods at one meal as this can challenge the digestive system.

Breakfast	Main Meal	Light Meal
A grain dish, such as waffles or granola. One or two pieces of fruit. Whole-grain bread and a fruit or nut spread.	A main course plus some raw vegetables (include a yellow and green vegetable if not already incorporated). Whole-grain bread with a fruit or protein spread.	A fruit dish, fresh fruit salad, or a light soup.

• As much as you can, choose foods that are
grown on healthy soils and eat them in or as
near to their natural state as possible.

The Lose–Fat Larder

Here is a brief guide to stocking a larder to give
you some idea of just how much variety you
have to choose from when you decide to Lose
Fat and Go Primitive.

Fruit

Not only are fruits some of the most delicious
natural foods available, they also have remarkable properties for spring cleaning the body
and are excellent biochemical antidotes to
stress.

Fruit contains very little protein but it is
very high in the mineral potassium, which
needs to be balanced with sodium for perfect
health in the body. Because most people in the
West eat far too much sodium in the form of
table salt and an excess of protein, eating good
quantities of fruit can help rebalance a body,
improve its functioning, and make you feel
more energetic as well.

Vegetables

The best vegetables are those you grow yourself organically. If you are lucky enough to have a garden—even a small one—save all the leftovers and turn them into compost for fertilizer. Even in winter you can grow some delicious salads and root vegetables in a greenhouse.

Scrubbing vegetables is better than peeling since many of the valuable vitamins and minerals are stored directly beneath their skins. Never soak vegetables for long periods. They are better washed briefly under running water so you don't allow water-soluble vitamins to leach out of them. Always keep vegetables as cool as possible (even carrots and turnips are best kept in the fridge) and use them as soon as you can.

Grains

Making sure a good portion of what you eat comes from grain foods—because of the effect on the brain of the complex carbohydrates they contain—tends to improve your disposition, making you feel calm and bringing you energy that lasts and lasts. But it is only by cooking them (or by sprouting or soaking them) that you turn hard-to-digest starches into more easily digested sugars. All grains can be toasted lightly. This process, which is called dextrinizing, not only helps turn starches into natural sugars but also enhances the flavor and is particularly good if you want to use grains to make oatmeal or other hot breakfast cereals. The more variety the better since each grain boasts a different balance of essential minerals and micronutrients.

Oils

When you Go Primitive do not use oils, except a very small quantity of cold-pressed soy oil or extra virgin olive oil. In heat-processed oils usable fatty acids have been chemically changed into junk fats that can not only be actively harmful, but also actually block the uptake of fatty acids from the rest of your diet. Olive oil adds a distinctive flavor to salad dressings. It is quite heavy, though, and some people prefer a lighter oil. Sesame is lighter and delicious, too. Cold-pressed walnut oil, if you can get it, is delicious for salads and full of essential fatty acids, but it is expensive and must be kept in the fridge.

Nuts

Quickstart does not use nuts. When buying
nuts for Living Lean make sure they are really
fresh. It is a good idea to buy a few different
kinds—mixing them will provide a good balance of essential amino acids.

Seeds

Except for a smattering of sesame seeds and
crushed linseeds Quickstart does not use seeds
either. During the Living Lean phase of Go
Primitive, be sure you buy really fresh seeds
with no signs of decay. The three seeds that
provide a valuable combination of protein and
essential fatty acids are sunflower, pumpkin,
and sesame.

Beans and legumes

Beans and legumes are rich in complex
carbohydrates, protein, and fiber as well as
minerals and essential fatty acids. All beans
and legumes should be washed and picked
over; then everything except lentils, split peas,
and mung beans should be soaked for at least
four to six hours before cooking. The soaking
water should then be thrown away and fresh

water added. When cooking beans and legumes there are two ways to minimize later digestive upset. The first is, after soaking and rinsing, to put them in the freezer overnight and cook the next day. The second is, after soaking, to throw the soaking water away, boil up the beans for 20 minutes, throw the first boil water away, rinse, then bring to a boil in fresh water and simmer until tender. Sprouting is another method, and the most nutritious by far.

Sprouts

Seeds and grains are latent powerhouses of nutritional goodness and life energy. Add water to germinate them, let them grow for a few days, and you will harvest delicious, inexpensive fresh foods of quite phenomenal health-enhancing value. Sprouts are, in effect, predigested. As such, they have many times the nutritional efficiency of the seeds from which they have grown. They provide more nutrients gram for gram than any natural food known.

Special foods

Carob (St. John's Bread). Carob powder/flour is a superb chocolate substitute—and good for you, too. Unlike chocolate it does not contain caffeine.

Agar-agar. This starch comes from seaweed. You can use it to make vegetarian gelatin-based sweets and salads and to thicken sauces and topping. It comes in flakes or granules and sometimes in sheets. Soak the agar-agar in a little arrowroot.

Arrowroot. Arrowroot is a nutritious, easily digested food high in calcium. When you heat it in water it thickens (use $1^1/_2$ teaspoons per cup of liquid). It is better than cornstarch or corn flour to thicken gravy, fruit sauces, soups, and stews.

Low-salt vegetable bouillon powder. This is something I use a lot to season just about everything.

Miso. A fermented soybean paste that is rich in digestive enzymes and high in protein. It can be used for seasoning soups and sauces.

Sea vegetables. If you have never used the sea vegetables for cooking, this is an ideal time to begin. Not only are they delicious—imparting a wonderful, spicy flavor to soups and salads—

they are also the richest source of organic mineral salts in nature, particularly of iodine. Sea vegetables are available in health-food stores and in Asian food shops. Recommended ones include the following:

arame	kombu
dulse	laver bread
hijiki	nori
kelp	wakami

Soy flour. Made from cooked, ground soybeans, soy flour is sometimes added to grain-based flours to increase their protein content. It can be used to make soy milk.

Soy milk. Made from cooked, ground, and strained soybeans, this is often used for bottle-fed infants who are allergic to cow's milk. I use it as a substitute for milk on cereals and in recipes.

Tahini (preferably unroasted). A paste made from ground sesame seeds that is tasty and very nutritious.

Tamari. This is a type of soy sauce made from fermented soybeans, but unlike soy sauce it contains no wheat, although it does contain sea salt, and so should be used in moderation.

Tofu. Its other name is bean curd. This white, bland, soft food made from soybeans is easy to digest, high in protein, low in calories and fat, cheap, and can be used for just about anything.

Yeast extract. This can be used as a substitute for vegetable bouillon. It is rich in B-complex vitamins but very salty, so it should be used in moderation.

RECIPES

Most of these recipes are designed to feed four people. And for reference, an ordinary cup holds about 8 fl oz (225 ml).

Breakfast

Breakfast is the most important meal of the day—between one-third and one-half of your calories should come from breakfast alone. A hearty breakfast full of complex carbohydrates

provides you with nutrient-rich fuel to keep
you going for 5 or 6 hours. Remember to drink
a couple of glasses of pure water as soon as you
wake up.

Feather–light waffles

  2 cups rolled oats
  3 tablespoons shredded coconut (optional)
$1/2$ teaspoon ground coriander
$1/2$ teaspoon cinnamon or nutmeg
  2 cups soy milk
  2 teaspoons vanilla essence
    pinch of salt

Heat up a nonstick waffle iron. Blend all the
ingredients together until creamy. Pour in
enough waffle mixture to cover the iron and
shut the lid. Leave to cook (without opening)
until the waffle stops steaming—about 7–10
minutes.
  Serve with a fruit topping or fresh fruit, or
mash a very ripe banana with a little concentrated fruit juice and spread it on.

Munchy–crunchy granola

An excellent make-it-ahead dried cereal that
you can keep in the fridge for instant break-

fast. It uses a mixture of grains. For Quick-start, omit the seeds since they are high in fat.

    5 cups steel-cut or rolled oats
    1 cup oat bran
    1 cup barley flakes
    1 cup wheat flakes
 $1/2$ cup rye flakes
 $1/2$ cup sunflower seeds
 $1/2$ cup raw sesame seeds
 $1/2$ cup sliced almonds
    2 cups pitted dates
$1^1/2$ cups fruit juice concentrate or 12 oz
        (300 g) can unsweetened concentrated
        pineapple juice
    1 tablespoon ground cinnamon
    2 teaspoons freshly grated nutmeg
    1 teaspoon ground coriander
    2 cups shredded, unsweetened coconut
    1 teaspoon salt
    1 cup raisins

Mix the grains, seeds, and almonds together. Place the dates, fruit juice, and all the other ingredients except the raisins in a food processor and mix until creamy. Add the fruit cream to the dry ingredients and mix with your hands in a large bowl. Spread the mixture on 3 large baking sheets, about 1 inch (2.5 cm)

thick, and put into a 325°F (170°C) oven. Cook
for 2 to 3 hours, stirring every half hour. After
the granola has cooled, mix in the raisins.
Store in airtight containers in a cool place.

Main Meals

These recipes are designed to form the core of a
main meal, which is best eaten at lunchtime or
before 4 o'clock in the afternoon when your
body handles energy most efficiently without
turning it into fat.

Serve your main dish together with a good
salad or a bowl of sprouted seeds and grains,
and some whole-grain bread. Do include green
vegetables, either in the salad or as cooked
vegetables.

Scrambled tofu

Scrambled tofu is great on whole-grain rye
toast. It is an excellent alternative to
scrambled eggs for Sunday brunch.

$^1/_2$ cup diced onions
$^1/_2$ cup diced carrots
$^1/_2$ cup chopped celery
  2 cloves garlic

1 teaspoon olive or soy oil

2 cups mashed, drained tofu

1 tablespoon low-salt vegetable bouillon
  powder or food yeast

1 teaspoon mild curry powder

Sauté onions, carrots, celery, and garlic in a
heavy frying pan using the olive or soy oil.
When brown, add the tofu, low-salt vegetable
bouillon, and curry powder. Stir together over
a medium heat for 5–10 minutes. Delicious
served with cottage fried potatoes (see page 66).

Luscious lentil soup

This soup is not really a soup at all but a
main course. It, like many of the soups I like
best, is like gruel—enormously nourishing
after long walks in the hills or on a dark winter's day.

14 oz (400 g) dried lentils

4 medium carrots, chopped

6 sticks celery, chopped

7 oz (200 g) small white potatoes, halved
  lengthwise

2–3 leeks, the white part

1 large onion, chopped

3–4 chopped tomatoes or a small can of
  tomatoes

 1 tablespoon black molasses (unsulfured)
 2 parsnips, chopped
 2–3 tablespoons low-salt vegetable bouillon
    powder
 ½ teaspoon dried sage
 ½ teaspoon dried thyme
 4 cloves garlic, crushed
    freshly ground black pepper
    juice of half a lemon
    freshly chopped parsley

Wash the lentils, place in a large pot, and cover
with 2–3 inches (5–7.5 cm) of water. Bring to a
boil. Add the remaining ingredients (except
lemon juice and parsley) and simmer for 45
minutes. I generally bring the soup to a boil
and then put it into a warm oven and just let it
sit for 45 minutes. Add lemon juice and parsley
just before serving.

Chili

Chili is one of my favorite dishes. I like to
make it thick and eat it with slabs of rich dark
bread or corn bread. I also like to purée it and
use it the next day to make burgers.

 2 cups dried kidney beans
 3 garlic cloves, crushed

1/2 cup green peppers, chopped

1 small onion, chopped

2 teaspoons olive oil

4 sticks celery, chopped

3 tablespoons canned tomatoes

2 tablespoons low-salt vegetable bouillon powder

2 teaspoons cumin

1 tablespoon chili powder

3 sprigs fresh marjoram

3 tablespoons concentrated apple juice

1/2 cup tomato paste

2 tablespoons spring water

Soak the beans overnight, rinse, and drain. Put into a pan and cover with spring water—about 2 inches (5 cm) above the beans. Bring to a boil and simmer until tender. Sauté the garlic, peppers, and onion in the olive oil, then add the remaining ingredients and stir well. Add this mixture to the kidney beans when they are cooked, readjusting the water as necessary, and simmer for another hour. Serve hot with warmed chunks of bread.

Easy vegetable curry

This is simple, delicious, and yet it takes no more than 20–30 minutes to prepare. It is

just as good eaten on its own or with a light
salad for supper. In smaller quantities it can be
served as a side dish to go with a large salad.

1 large onion, finely chopped
1 teaspoon olive oil
2 teaspoons mild curry powder
1–1^1/$_2$ teaspoons low-salt vegetable bouillon
  powder
3 large carrots (cut in 1^1/$_2$-in sticks)
1 medium-sized turnip, cut into matchsticks
2 potatoes, cut into chunks
1^1/$_2$ cups spring water
  grated coconut (optional)

Sauté the onion in the oil until it becomes
translucent, then add the curry powder and
vegetable bouillon powder and continue to stir
for a few minutes. Add the rest of the vegetables and pour in the water. Bring to a boil
and simmer slowly for 20–30 minutes, then
serve. It is particularly nice served with some
grated dried coconut.

This vegetable curry can be adapted to whatever vegetables you have on hand. During the
summer it's delightful to be able to add some
green beans or perhaps some peas, or chopped
celery.

Burgers

I adore putting burgers together with Go Primitive ingredients and stacking them high on whole-grain hamburger buns full of tomato slices, pimento cheese, and onions, and all the other condiments in their low-fat form.

    4 whole-grain hamburger buns, halved
    1 cup tofu mayonnaise (see page 71)
    4 burgers (see burger mix, below)
    4 thick slices tomato
    4 slices red onion
    4 lettuce leaves
  3/4 cup alfalfa sprouts (optional)

Spread the buns lavishly with the mayonnaise and layer the other ingredients, including the burgers, on top to make as thick a sandwich as you can manage and still get your teeth round it—my number one favorite.

Burger mix

You can make burgers from just about any leftover legumes that you have—lima beans, black-eyed peas, kidney beans, or chickpeas. Here's how.

2 cups mashed beans or legumes
2 tablespoons chickpea flour or fine wheat
   flour
1 onion, minced
2 tablespoons low-salt vegetable bouillon
   powder
2 tablespoons Worcestershire sauce
2 cloves garlic, crushed or finely chopped
1 teaspoon sage
1 cup breadcrumbs, seasoned

Blend the cooked beans or legumes until smooth. Pour into a bowl and add the other ingredients (except the breadcrumbs). Shape into patties. Roll in seasoned breadcrumbs and either bake for 45 minutes in a 375°F (190°C) oven or cook in a nonstick frying pan until golden brown on both sides.

Pizza

This is a basic recipe for a pizza that you can, of course, adapt as you like. There are so many delicious toppings you could go on experimenting forever.

Pizza base:
1 tablespoon yeast

1 cup spring water (warmed to activate the
  yeast)
3 cups finely ground wheat flour
1 teaspoon salt

Stir the yeast into the water and allow to
stand for 15 minutes until the water has a thin
layer of bubbles. Add the yeast mixture to the
flour and salt and knead (in a processor if you
can) until you have a firm ball. Knead for
another 10 minutes by hand, adding more flour
if the dough is too sticky. Put the dough in a
bowl draped with a clean dishcloth and leave
in a warm place for 45 minutes, or until the
dough has doubled in size. Push it back down
to get rid of some of the air and knead again
for just 1 minute. Pull the dough out into a
circle with your fingers, making sure it is
thicker at the edges than in the middle.
Lightly flour a baking tray and put the pizza
base on it.

Pizza sauce:
  1 cup tomato purée
  ½ cup apple concentrate
    juice of 1 lemon
  2 teaspoons low-salt vegetable bouillon
    powder
  1 clove garlic, crushed

$1/4$ teaspoon oregano
1 teaspoon salt

Make your pizza sauce by putting all the ingredients in a food processor and blending well. If it is too thick add a little water. Spread the sauce over the uncooked pizza base and add a topping (see below).

Pizza topping:
Once your pizza sauce is made, choose your toppings from the list below.

1 cup mushrooms
2 large tomatoes, sliced
    a handful of pitted olives
1 green pepper, sliced
1 yellow pepper, sliced
1 red pepper, sliced
2 cloves garlic, cut into slivers
1 red onion, finely sliced
4–5 fresh basil leaves, finely chopped
$1/2$ teaspoon oregano
$1/2$ teaspoon thyme
    freshly ground black pepper

Arrange your choice of topping over the pizza base, adding anything else your imagination inspires you to use. Place in a hot oven and cook for 15 minutes or until the crust has browned. Serve piping hot from the oven or eat cold.

Grains

Here are some grain dishes that can themselves be the basis of a main meal served together with a salad or vegetables. Grains are particularly good for athletes since they are the lightest form of complex carbohydrates to release energy slowly over many hours while you work or exercise. Each grain has its own natural characteristic. The important thing is to vary the grains that you eat, for each grain also has its own synergistic complements of vitamins and minerals.

Yummy brown rice

1 cup brown rice
2–3 cups spring water
2 teaspoons low-salt vegetable bouillon
  powder
1 teaspoon marjoram
2 cloves garlic, finely chopped (optional)
3 tablespoons fresh parsley, chopped

Wash the rice three times under running water
and put into a saucepan. Boil the water in a
kettle and pour over the rice. Add seasonings
except for the parsley. Bring to a boil and cook
gently for 45 minutes or until all the liquid has
been absorbed. Garnish with parsley and
serve. If you double the quantities used here
you can keep some and make a delicious rice
salad the next day.

Barley pilaf

A delicious baked dish. It is made from pot
barley, not from pearl barley. Barley is also
excellent used in soups.

      2 onions, finely chopped
      1 teaspoon olive oil
      1 cup pot barley
  1½ cups spring water
      1 tablespoon low-salt vegetable bouillon
         powder
      1 tablespoon dill
      2 cloves garlic, finely chopped (optional)

Sauté the onions in the oil until translucent,
then add the barley to the pan and stir well.
Remove from the heat and add the remaining
ingredients (including the water, boiled in a

kettle). Place in a lightly oiled oven dish and bake in a moderate oven for half an hour. Check to see if you need to add a little more water. Serve immediately.

Vegetables

Vegetables have become the most neglected of all natural foods in the last half-century and it is a pity because the color, texture, and variety of flavors they offer is quite remarkable. As you vary the grains, try also to vary the vegetables. The best way to cook vegetables is either to steam them or to wok fry them in a teaspoon of olive or sesame oil. Don't overcook them or you will ruin their flavor and cause them to lose their color.

Baked carrots

  6 large carrots
  1 teaspoon olive oil
 $1/4$ cup sesame seeds

Scrub the carrots well and slice them lengthwise 4 or 5 times, then crosswise into pieces about 3 inches (7.5 cm) long. Mix well with the oil, then place on a baking sheet and bake in a hot oven for 20 minutes. During the last 10 minutes of baking sprinkle the sesame seeds over the top. Serve immediately.

Cottage fried potatoes

These are a great replacement for chips or French fries. Kids love them.

6 medium potatoes
1 tablespoon garlic salt
1 tablespoon onion salt
2 tablespoons finely milled whole-grain flour

Scrub the potatoes thoroughly, leaving the skins on. Cut them lengthwise in strips or put them through a food processor using the chipper attachment. Mix the garlic salt and onion salt with the flour. Sprinkle over the potatoes (their dampness will pick up a fine coating of the flour mixture). Place on a non-stick baking sheet and bake for 30–40 minutes at 450°F (230°C).

Baked parsnips

The sweetness of parsnips always surprises me. Full of fiber and delicious, they are one of my favorite vegetables. This is an easy way to get the best from them.

14 oz (400 g) fresh parsnips
 3 tablespoons concentrated fruit juice or
   1 teaspoon olive oil
1/2 teaspoon low-salt vegetable bouillon
   powder
 2 tablespoons Dijon mustard

Slice the parsnips lengthwise 2 or 3 times, then crosswise into lengths about 3 inches (7.5 cm) long. Mix together the fruit concentrate or oil, the vegetable bouillon powder, and the mustard, and pour over to cover the parsnips using a tablespoon or two of water in the mixture if you need it. Bake in a moderate oven until golden brown—about 30–35 minutes.

Salads

These salads can be substantial whole meals, and one way of making an excellent whole-meal salad is with leftover grains or beans from the day before, mixed together with every variety of raw vegetables. They bring to the

table a burst of fresh and vibrant color and
wonderful crunchy flavor.

Italian salad

The Italians make some of the most delicious
salads of all because they grow such splendid
vegetables. When I visit Italy I buy several
packets of seeds to grow different types of lettuce and basil in the garden.

1 head Italian red lettuce (radicchio)
1 small head romaine lettuce, finely shredded
1 red pepper, cut into rings
1 yellow pepper, cut into rings
1–2 large Italian tomatoes, sliced
4 radishes, chopped
  a few button mushrooms, finely sliced
1 teaspoon fennel seeds
1 red onion, cut into thin rings

Make a nest of the 2 shredded lettuces in
a shallow dish and arrange the other vegetables in the center, sprinkling the onion on
the top.

Apple ginger salad

Another very simple salad that goes with almost any dish. The ginger is a natural digestion aid.

  6 green apples
 1/4 cup fresh orange juice
  1 teaspoon fresh ginger, grated
  2 teaspoons clear honey (optional)
  3 tablespoons sesame seeds, toasted

Quarter the apples, remove the cores, and then finely slice by hand or in a processor. Combine the orange juice, ginger, and honey, and pour over the apples immediately to prevent them going brown. Add the toasted sesame seeds and toss well.

Bulgur salad with endive

A delicious and substantial dish that, thanks to the endive and the bulgur wheat, is high in vitamin E.

1 lb (450 g) bulgur wheat, cooked
  2 endives
 10 scallions
     a bunch of watercress

For the dressing:

3 tablespoons fresh lemon juice
1 tablespoon low-salt vegetable bouillon
   powder
1 teaspoon balsamic vinegar
3 cloves garlic, crushed
1 tablespoon Dijon mustard
1 teaspoon dried tarragon leaf
   pinch of salt and freshly ground black pepper

Soak the bulgur wheat overnight or for at least
3 hours in enough water to cover. Then drain
excess water and place in a bowl. Put the
ingredients for the dressing into a screw-top
jar and shake well until mixed. Add endives,
scallions, and watercress to the bulgur wheat
and mix. Pour the dressing over the salad
and toss.

Sauces and Spreads

These recipes add extra flavor and texture to
grain dishes, to vegetables, and to salads, but
some are so delicious you could eat them on
their own or dip crunchy toast into them.
Experiment with sauces and spreads to see

what wonderful concoctions you can come
up with.

Tofu mayonnaise

2 cups tofu
2 cloves garlic
   juice of 3 lemons
1 tablespoon low-salt vegetable bouillon
   powder
2 teaspoons curry powder
2 teaspoons onion powder
   pinch of salt

Put all the ingredients in a food processor and
blend until smooth. If it is too thick, add a little
water.

Tomato vinaigrette

This vinaigrette is particularly good on a green
salad.

2/3 cup tomato juice
  1 tablespoon balsamic vinegar
  2 cloves garlic, crushed
  1 teaspoon onion salt
 10 leaves fresh basil or tarragon

pinch of salt
black pepper to taste

Blend all ingredients in a food processor, then season to taste.

Eggplant pâté

You can vary the taste of eggplant pâté considerably by adding different spices or different extra ingredients but the principles of making it are simple. You must make sure you puncture the skins of the eggplants before baking as they will explode—this happened to me once and it blew the oven door open.

2 medium eggplants
4 cloves garlic, finely chopped
4 tablespoons fresh parsley, finely chopped
1 small onion, finely chopped
   juice of 1–2 lemons
1/2 cup tahini
1 teaspoon low-salt vegetable bouillon
   powder or other seasoning
1/2 teaspoon ground cumin
   pinch of cayenne

Remove the stems from the eggplants and prick them with a fork as you would a potato.

Put them into the oven and bake slowly for about 30 minutes until they become soft inside. Remove them and, being careful not to burn your fingers, scoop out the inner flesh, tossing the skins away. Put into a food processor to purée. Combine all the other ingredients in the food processor with the purée, remove, and chill in the fridge.

Mock guacamole

If you are a guacamole lover, as I am, but don't want to eat all the fat that comes with avocados, this is a great substitute.

   3 cups garden peas
   3 cloves garlic, crushed
   1 tablespoon low-salt vegetable bouillon
     powder
1/2 teaspoon chili powder
     juice of 2 lemons
     dash of Worcestershire sauce
   1 red onion, chopped finely

Steam the peas lightly, being careful not to cook them too much so that they keep their brilliant color. Purée everything but the chopped onion in a food processor, then add the chopped onion and mix well by hand. Chill and serve.

Raw hummus

This works well as a dressing but, if made with less liquid, is also delicious spread on bread or rice cakes.

2 cups sprouted chickpeas
   juice of 3 lemons
1 teaspoon low-salt vegetable bouillon powder
1 clove garlic, finely chopped
3 tablespoons scallions or chives, chopped

Put the ingredients (except the chives or scallions) into a food processor or blender and blend thoroughly. Then mix in the chopped chives or scallions and chill. This dressing will keep for 2 to 3 days in the fridge.

Desserts

One of the great pleasures of the Lose Fat scheme is being able to eat desserts again and know that all the pleasure you get from eating them will be echoed in the benefits that they can bring your body.

Pineapple blackberry frappé

This makes a wonderfully refreshing dessert as it stands, or can be chilled to serve as a cool sorbet on hot summer days.

  2 cups fresh pineapple chunks
$1/2$ cup blackberries
      juice of half a lime (optional)

Place all the ingredients in a blender and liquify. Serve immediately.

Apple bread pudding

Bread pudding is such a wonderful way of using practically any kind of stale bread. This works best with whole-wheat bread.

  2 cups soy milk or skim milk
$1/2$ cup concentrated apricot juice
  2 teaspoons vanilla essence
      pinch of salt
 12 slices bread, cubed
  4 medium apples
$1^1/2$ cups raisins
      juice of half a lemon
  1 teaspoon Amaretto
$1/4$ teaspoon freshly grated nutmeg

Mix the soy milk together with the apricot concentrate, vanilla essence, and salt. Tear the bread into small cubes and mash it into the milk mixture. Allow to soak for 15 minutes. In another bowl combine the apple, raisins, lemon juice, and Amaretto. Add to the bread mixture and toss gently. Pour into a nonstick baking pan, sprinkle with nutmeg, and cook in a preheated oven at 350°F (180°C) for 45 minutes or until set and browned on top. Serve warm.

Carob and banana ice cream

This recipe is one of my family favorites. The combination of carob and banana we find unbeatable.

  4 cups (about a quart or 2 pints) soy milk
  4 ripe bananas
  3 tablespoons granular lecithin (optional)
  1 cup unheated carob powder
  $1/2$ cup pear concentrate
  1 teaspoon vanilla essence

Freeze the milk in a low flat plastic container. Remove from the freezer and let it sit for about half an hour until it is just soft enough to slice into pieces. Put the bananas into the food processor, add about a cup of the frozen milk and the lecithin, carob powder, pear concentrate, and vanilla, and blend until just mixed. Add the remainder of the soy milk. (Don't overblend or you will make the ice cream too liquid. Should this happen, simply return it to the freezer for a few minutes, then stir before serving.) Serve immediately.

Further Reading

If you benefited from this book by health and beauty expert Leslie Kenton, you might like to try the entire series of quick and easy tips for living:

BEAT STRESS (8041-1626-1)
Discover how to identify, then eliminate everyday tension through relaxation, diet, and exercise.

BOOST ENERGY (8041-1625-3)
Increase your stamina and optimize your efficiency by changing your everyday routine.

GET FIT (8041-1628-8)
Develop the best exercise program for your lifestyle, and find out how to stick with it.

LOOK GREAT (8041-1623-7)
Learn the basics for making the most of your appearance by selecting, or creating, effective beauty products.

LOSE FAT (8041-1624-5)
Win the weight war through a simple eating plan that turns food into energy—not fat.

SLEEP DEEP (8041-1627-X)
Get the rest you need with relaxation techniques and healthy, natural sleep potions.

Index

DR. DEAN ORNISH'S PROGRAM
FOR REVERSING HEART DISEASE
by Dr. Dean Ornish

Dr. Dean Ornish is the first clinician to offer documented proof that heart disease can be halted or even reversed simply by changing your lifestyle. In this breakthrough book, he guides you step-by-step through the extraordinary Opening Your Heart Program that takes you beyond the purely physical side of health care to include the psychological, emotional, and spiritual aspects so vital to healing.

FOOD AND HEALING
by Annemarie Colbin

We must take responsibility for our own health and rely less on modern medicine, which seems to focus on trying to cure rather than prevent illness. Eating well is the first step toward better health and includes the latest information on new dietary systems, low-fat eating, food combining, and alternative medicine.

BETWEEN HEAVEN AND EARTH:
A Guide to Chinese Medicine
by Harriet Beinfield, L. Ac.,
and Efrem Korngold, L. Ac., O.M.D.
Pioneers in the practice of acupuncture and herbal medicine explain the philosophy behind Chinese medicine, how it works, and what it can do. Combining Eastern traditions with Western sensibilities in a unique blend that is relevant today, this book addresses three vital areas of Chinese medicine to present a comprehensive yet understandable guide to this ancient system.

NATURAL PRESCRIPTIONS
by Robert M. Giller, M.D.,
and Kathy Matthews
A natural treatment is the best kind—one that helps the body heal itself. Based on his years of practical experience as a doctor, as well as on the latest research, Dr. Giller's book explains in crystal-clear terms how to treat yourself with vitamin and mineral supplements, herbs, diet, exercise, and stress reduction.